MINDFULNESS

FOR

BEGINNERS

by

Dalida Turkovic

Print information available on the last page

Rev. date: 02/19/2016

To order additional copies of this book, contact:
Xlibris
1-888-795-4274
www.Xlibris.com
Orders@Xlibris.com

A heartfelt gratitude to: Nataly Ba, Anita and Dusan Mitrovic, Ann Marie McKelvey, Dhuruv Dev Singh, Mimi Pullen, Martin Barnes and all who encouraged me to keep drawing

Dedicated to
Jovan, Ivan and Boris

Once upon a time grownups
believed that Earth was flat

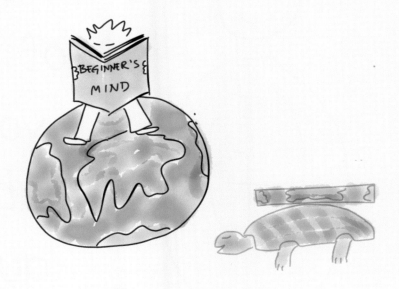

It is important to keep an open mind
for new ideas.

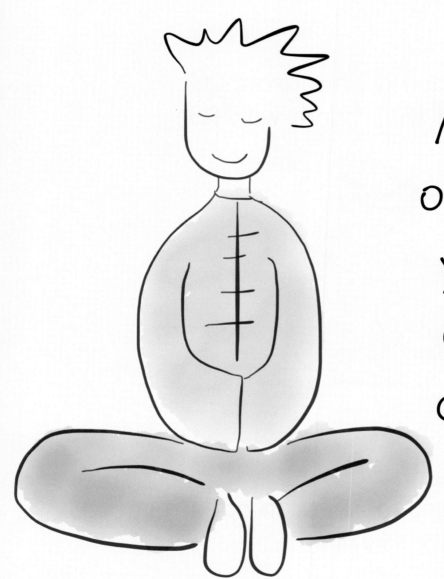

At the end of this book you will be able to sit quietly and observe...

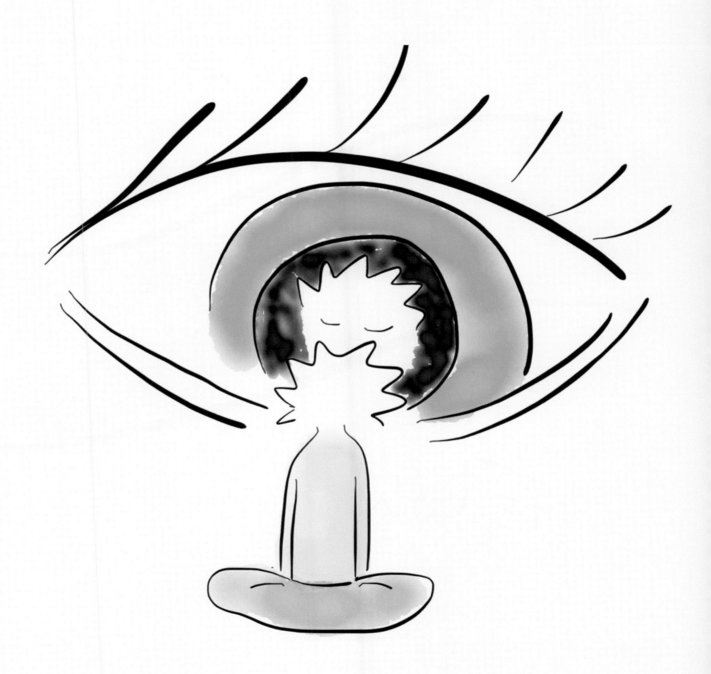

The
Flow

4

You know that feeling when you play and nothing really matters?

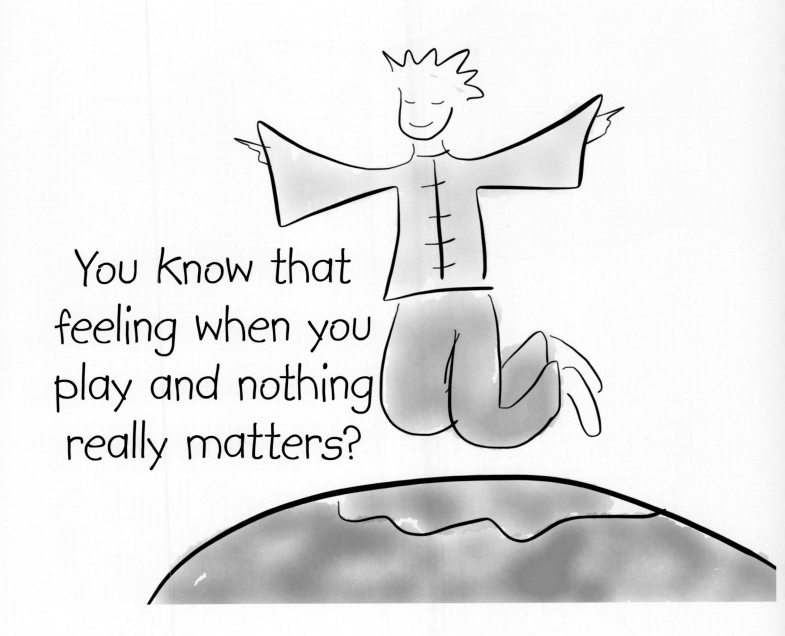

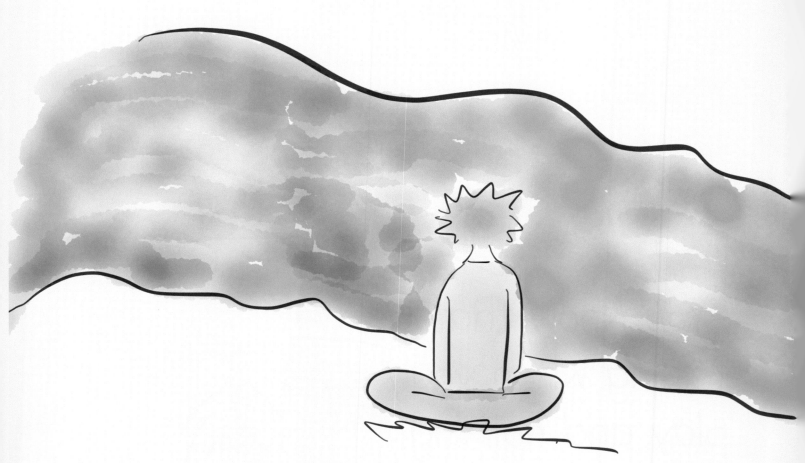

Grown ups call it the Flow and they get great results if they can feel it while they work or when doing any other activity.

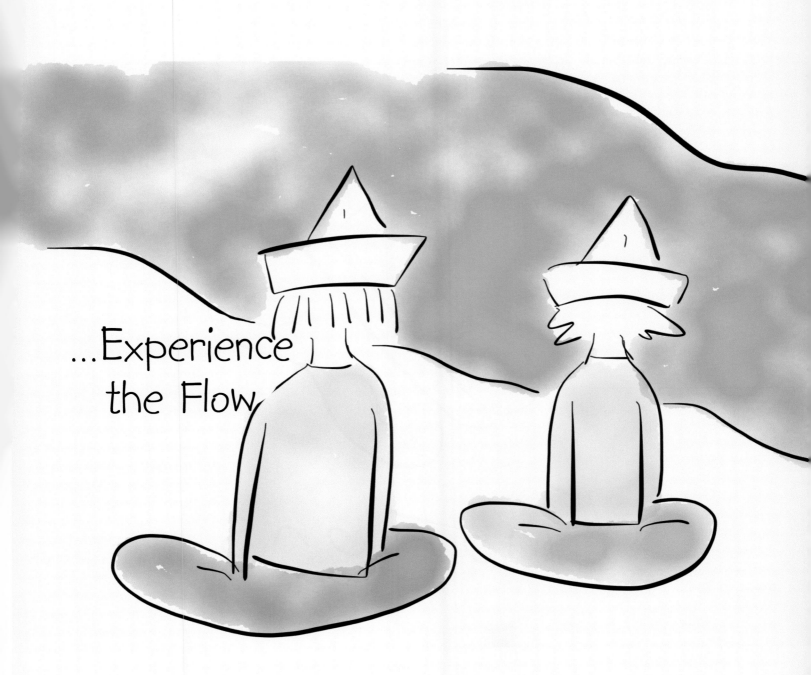

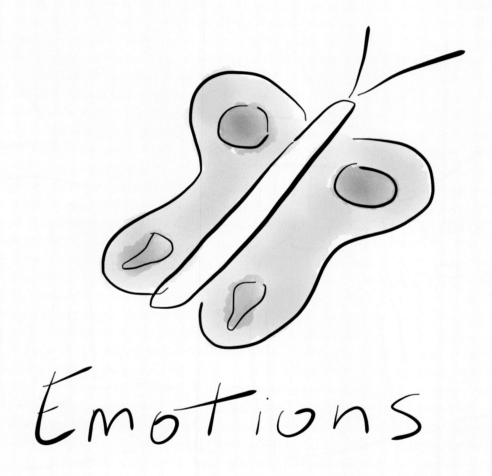

Emotions

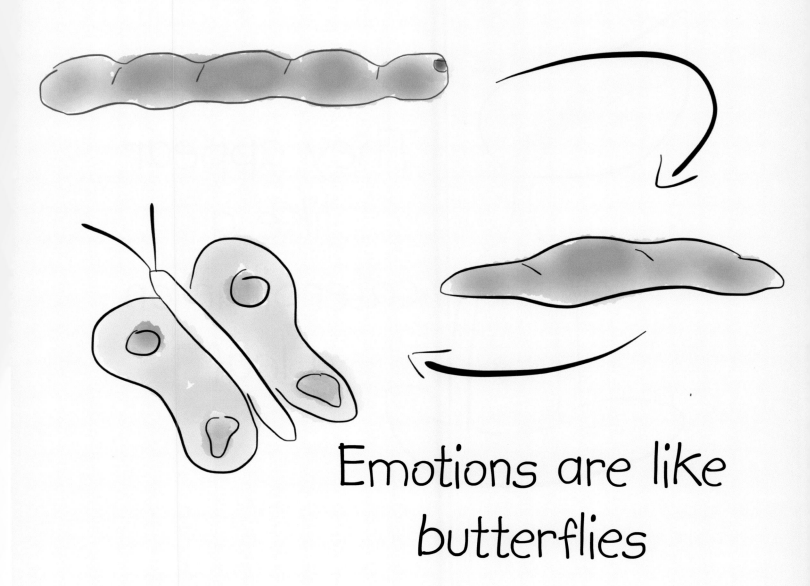

Emotions are like butterflies

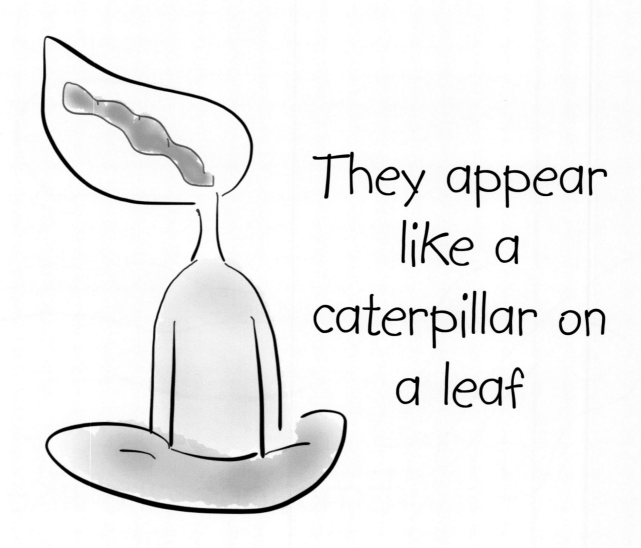

They appear like a caterpillar on a leaf

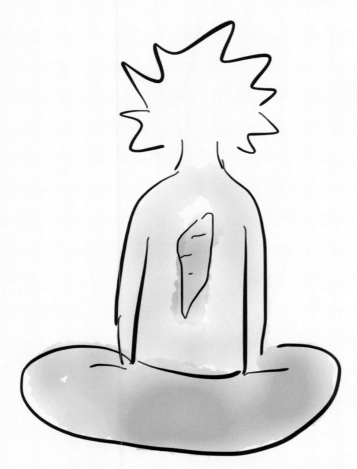

Observe where
they land in
your body...
like a cocoon
or a larva

Grown ups
can carry
emotions
for a long
time without
paying
attention

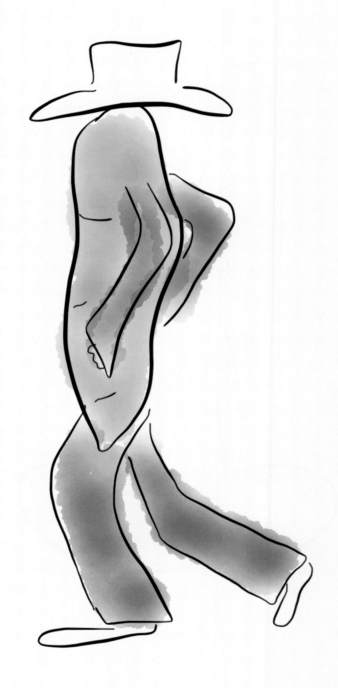

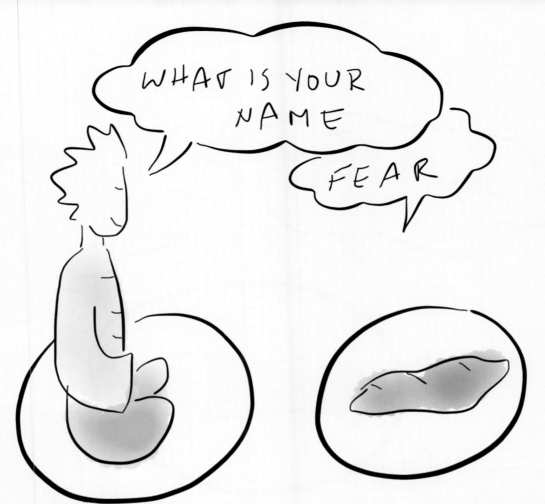

Instead of ignoring your emotions, treat them like a friend. Ask them politely what they want and what they need.

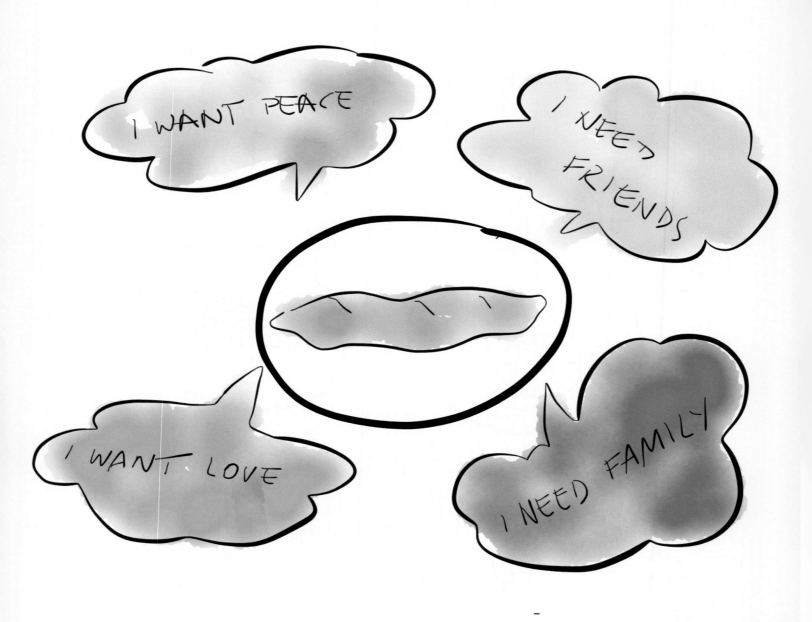

All you need to do is ask and listen...

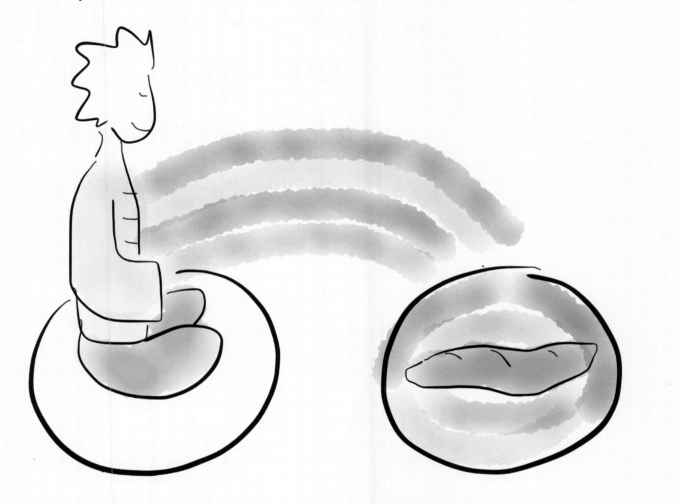

Give that emotion all it wants, give it what it needs.

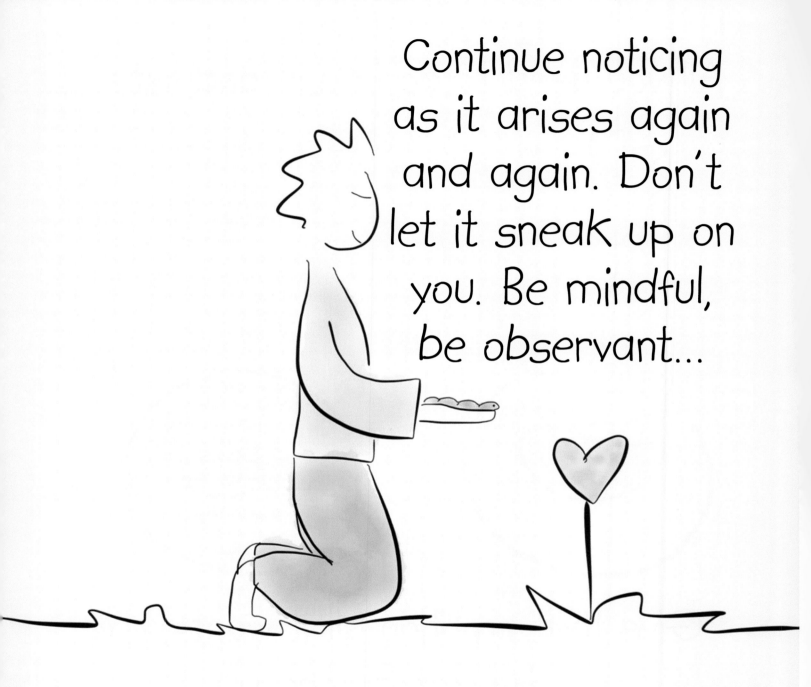

Continue noticing as it arises again and again. Don't let it sneak up on you. Be mindful, be observant...

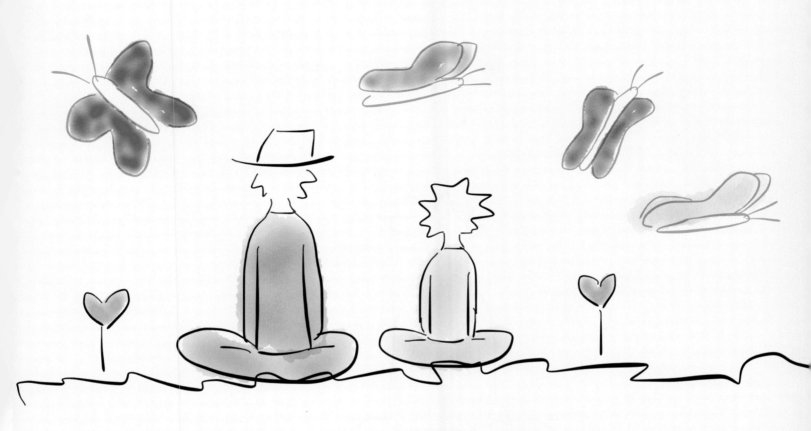

Emotions can be our friends.
They help us learn what we
want and what we need. They
help us grow.

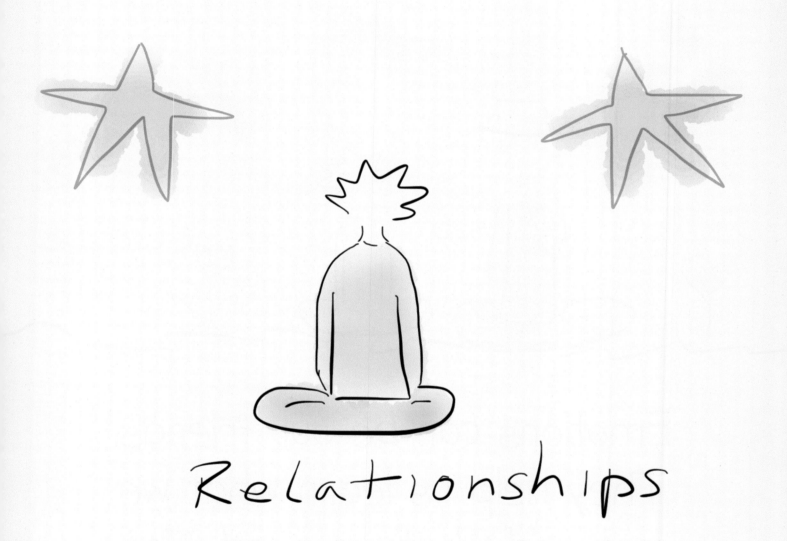

Relationships

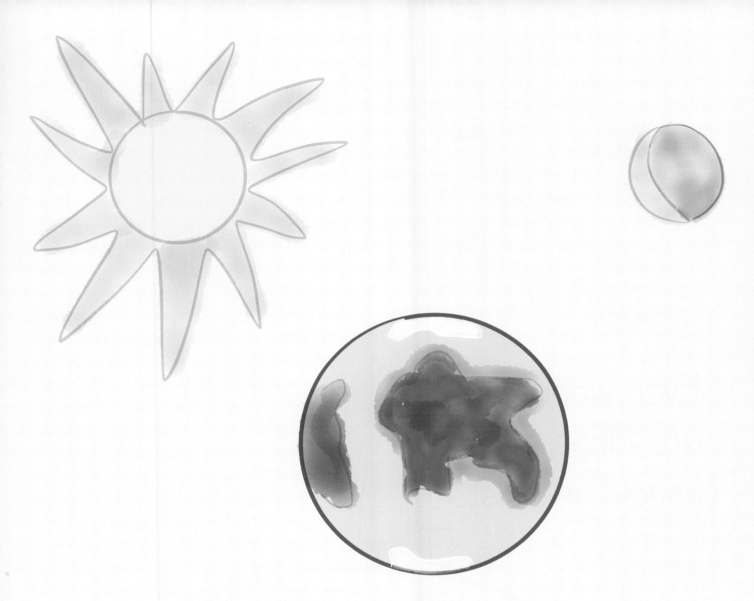

You and I are like a universe – we need each other and provide for each other like the Sun and the Moon do for Earth

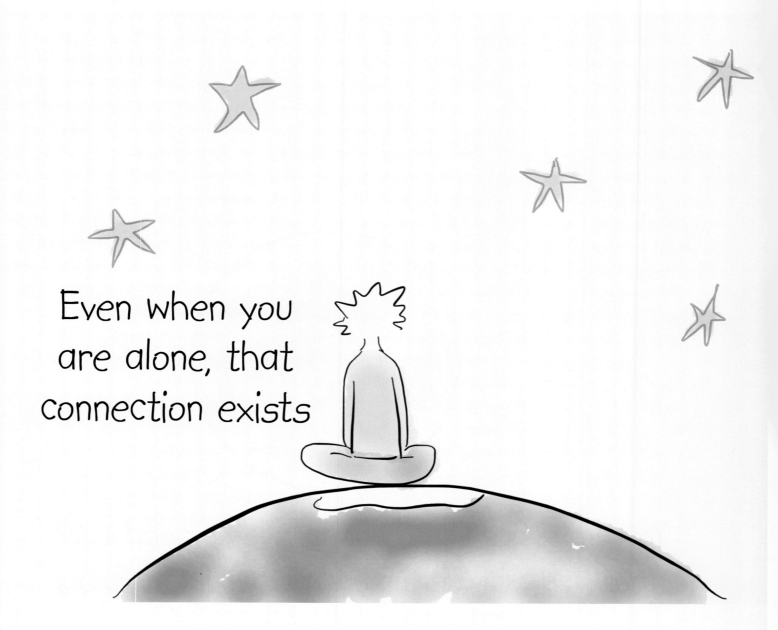

Even when you are alone, that connection exists

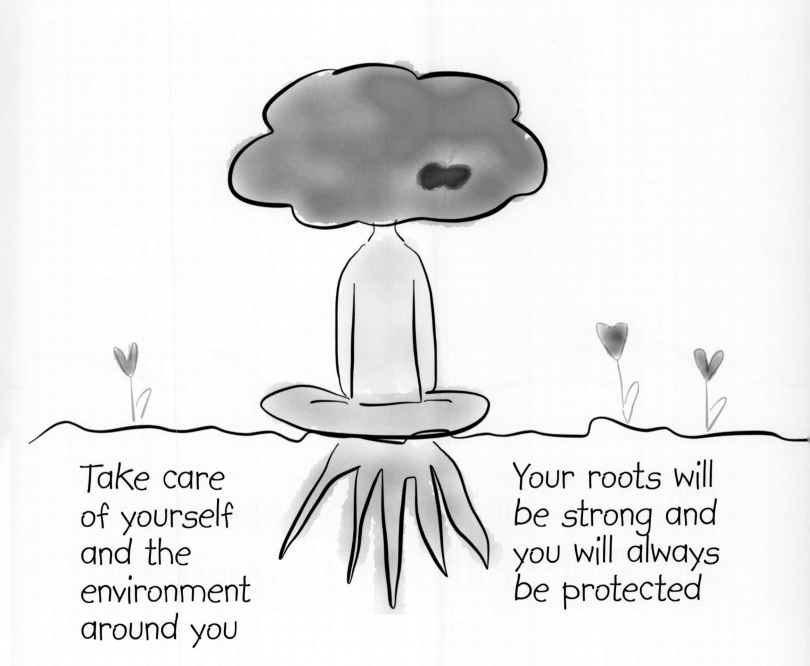

Take care
of yourself
and the
environment
around you

Your roots will
be strong and
you will always
be protected

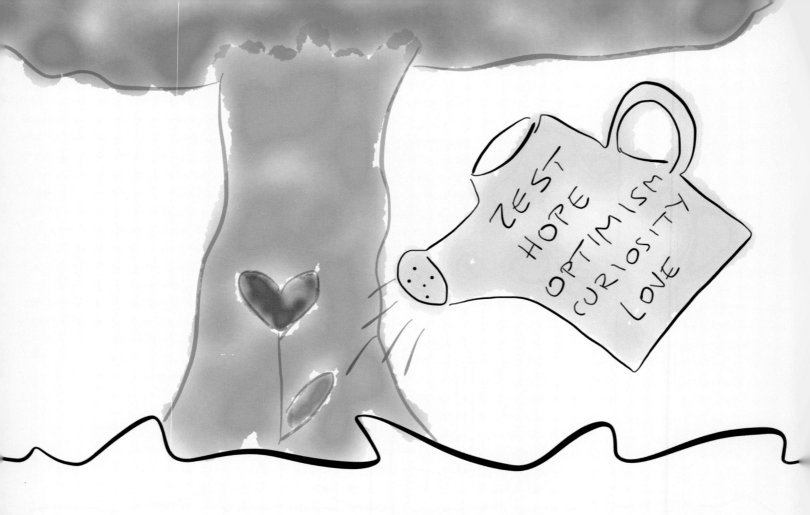

Fill your bucket with happiness
and share with others wherever
you are

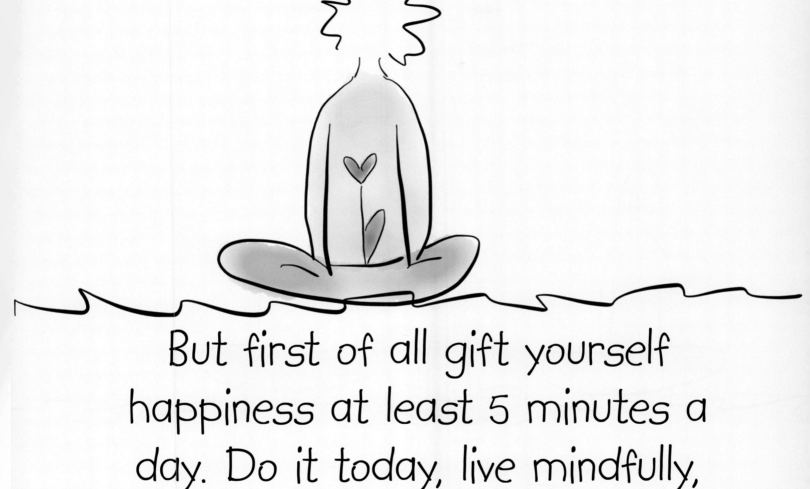

But first of all gift yourself
happiness at least 5 minutes a
day. Do it today, live mindfully,
celebrate life every step of
the Way!

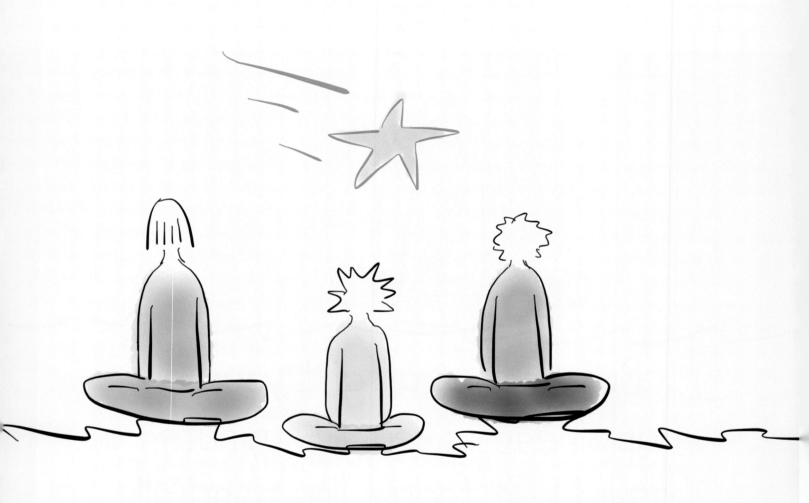

There are no
ordinary moments

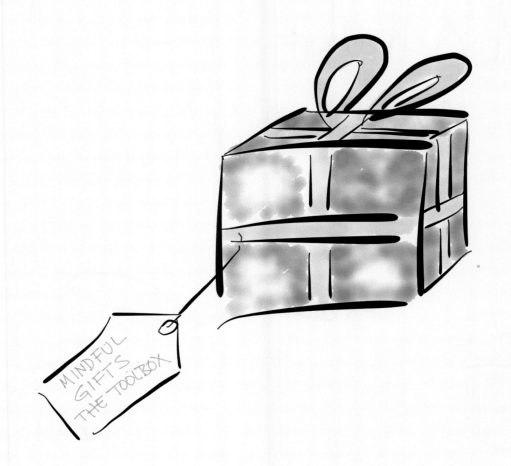

MINDFUL
GIFTS
THE TOOLBOX

Mindful Walking

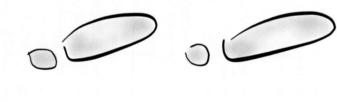

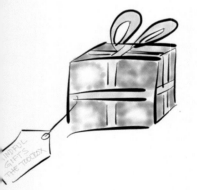

Small Steps

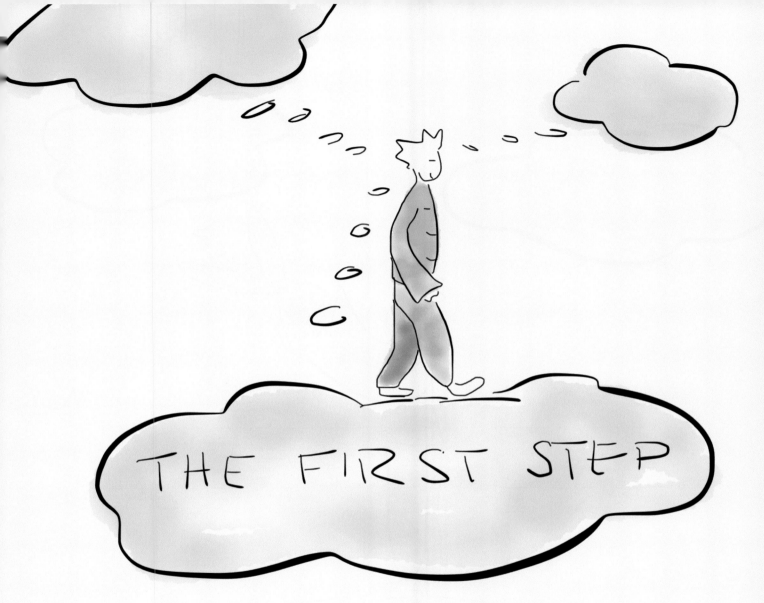

THE FIRST STEP

Notice at first... Your thoughts... they come & go

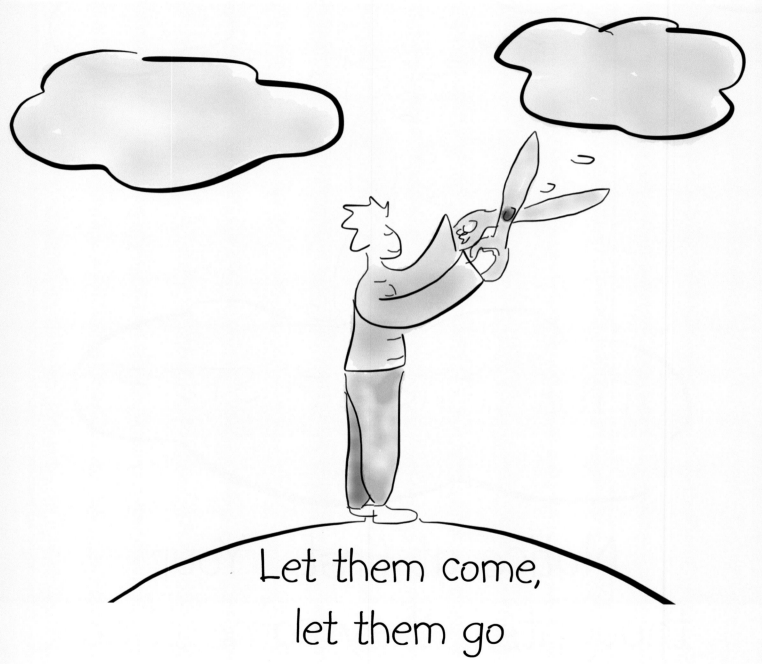

Let them come,
let them go

Find a spot
away from
distractions
and let your
awareness
sink into
your feet

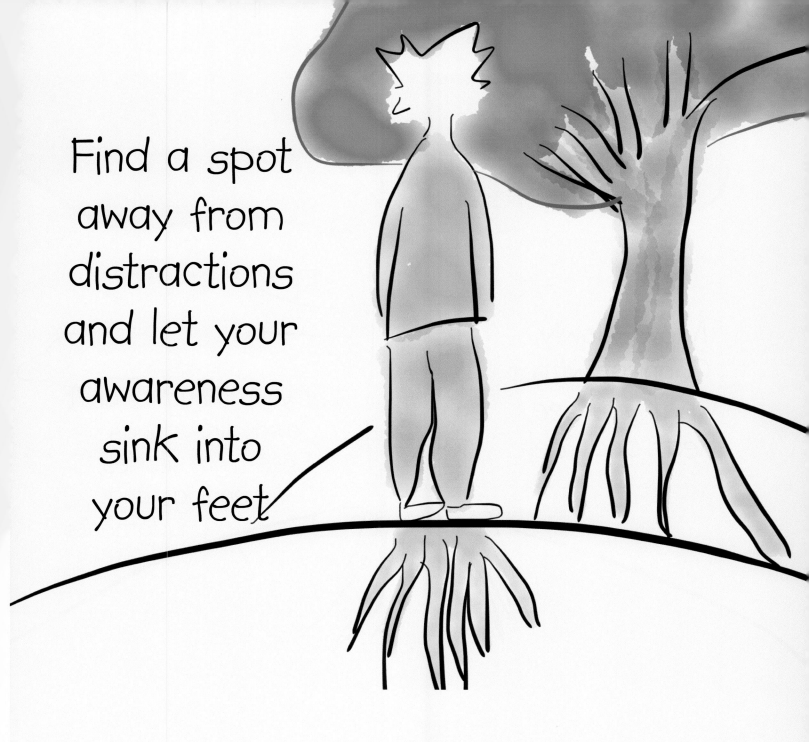

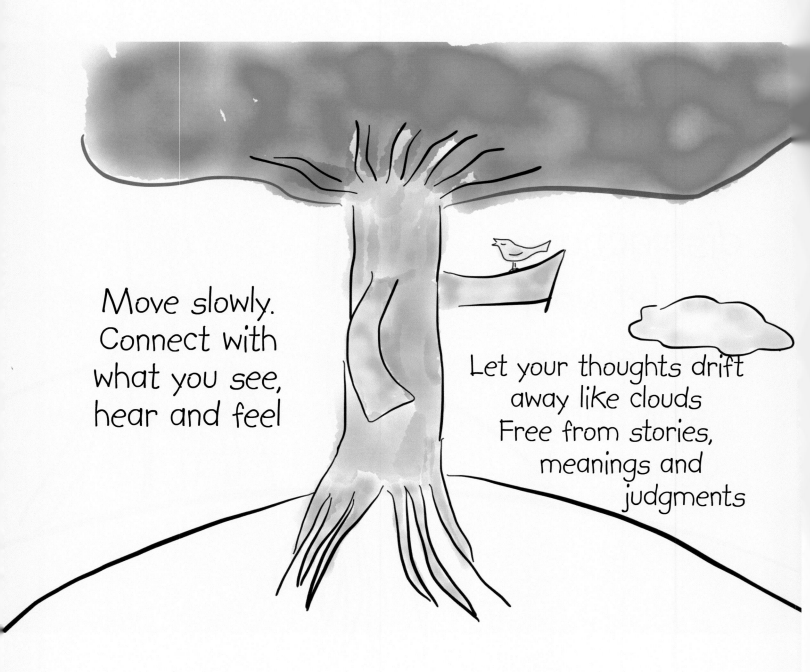

Move slowly.
Connect with
what you see,
hear and feel

Let your thoughts drift
away like clouds
Free from stories,
meanings and
judgments

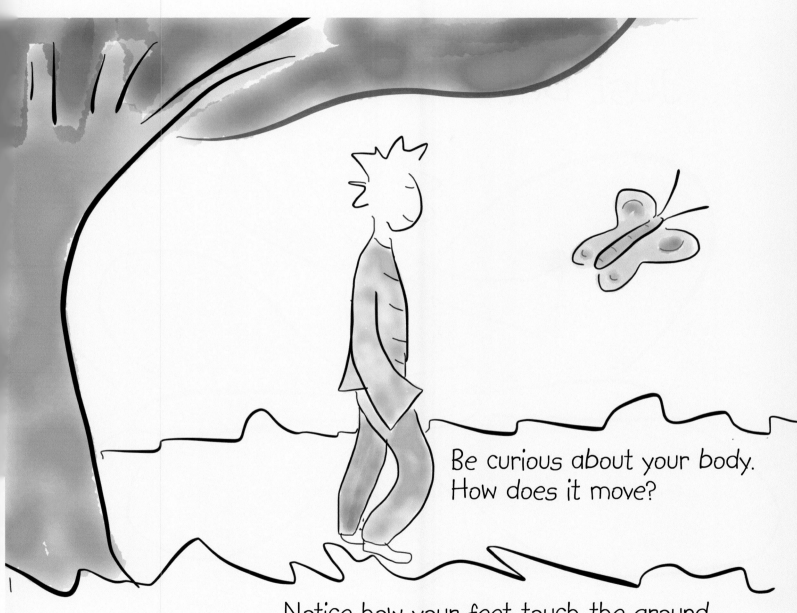

Be curious about your body.
How does it move?

Notice how your feet touch the ground...
move s-l-o-w-l-y... What do you notice?

Just be!

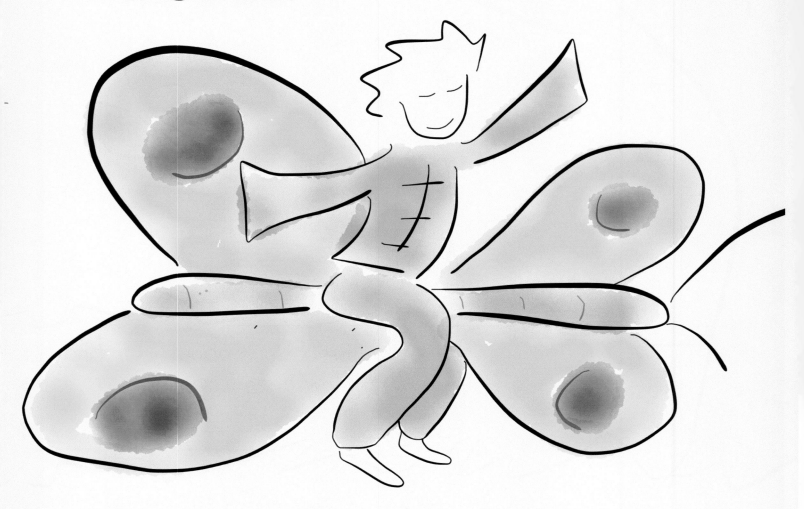

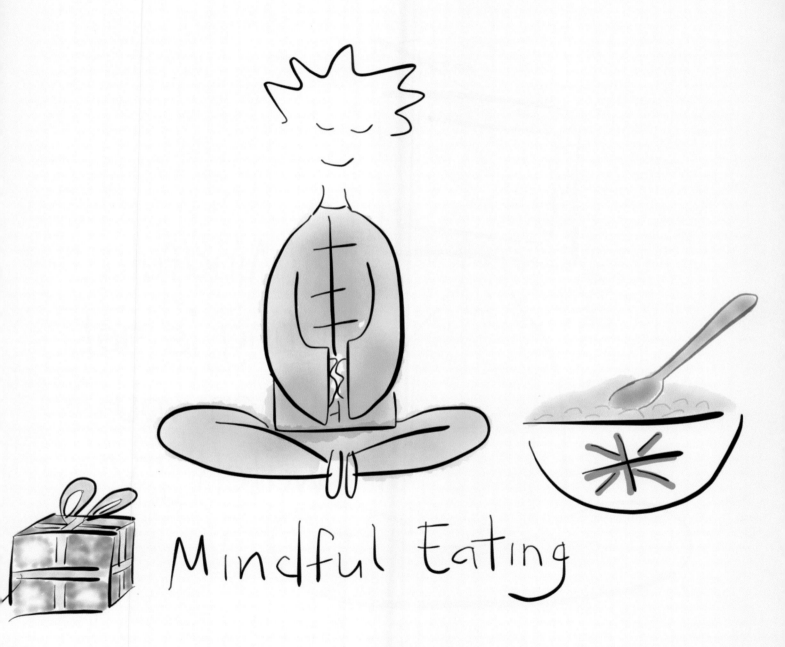

Mindful Eating

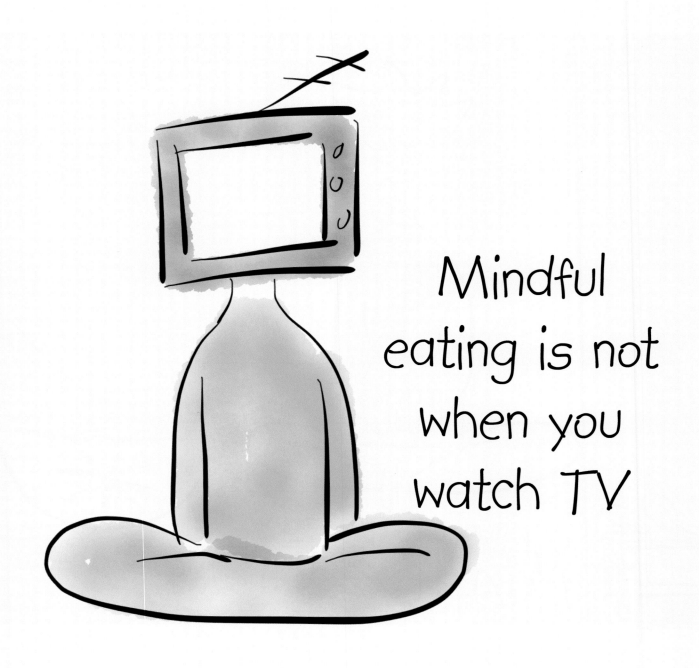

Mindful eating is not when you watch TV

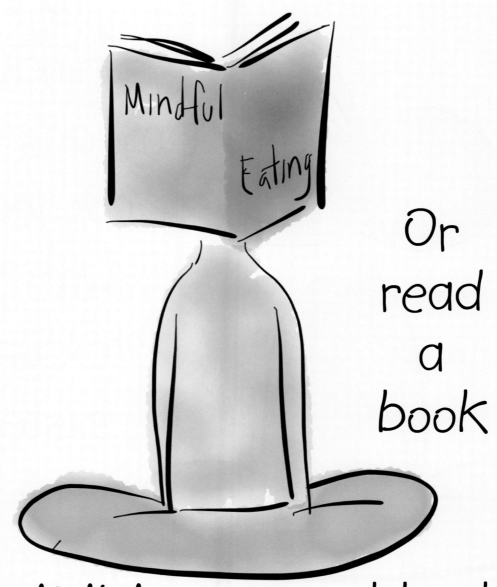

Or
read
a
book

Even if it is ... a cookbook...

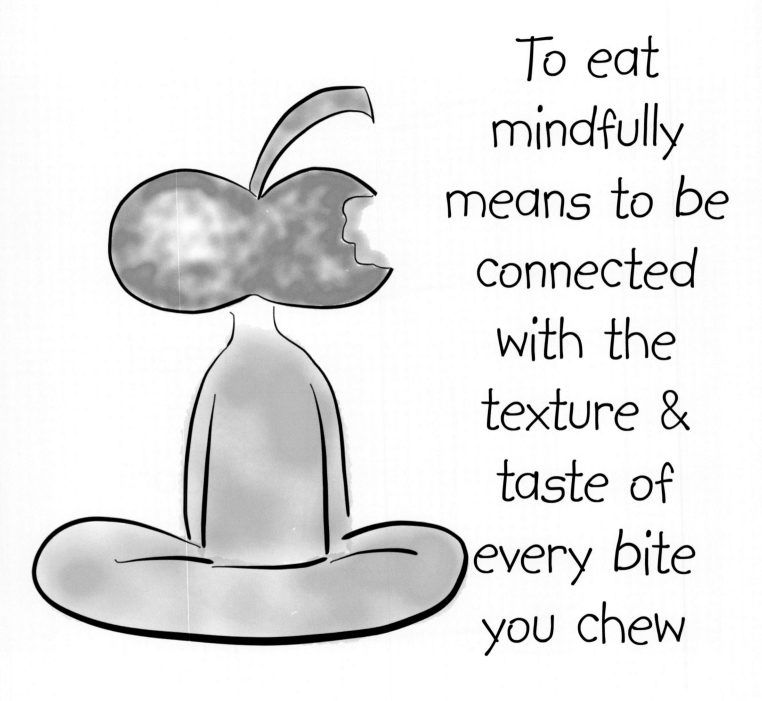

To eat mindfully means to be connected with the texture & taste of every bite you chew

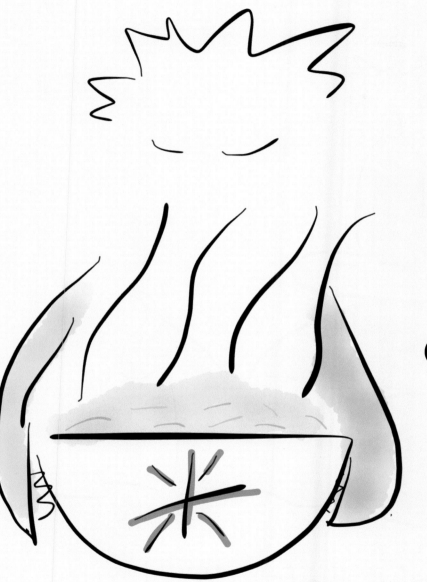

Experience
the smell
and warmth
of your
nutritious
food

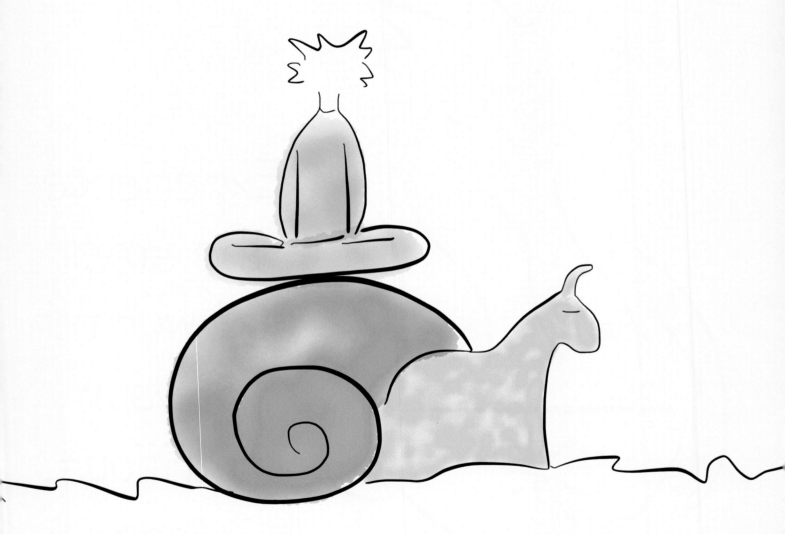

Once again, take it slow...

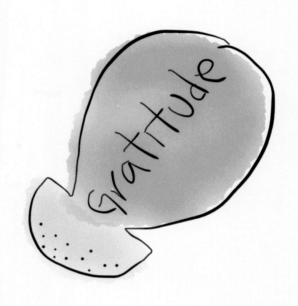

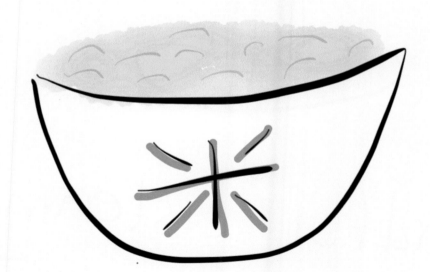

And spice it up with gratitude

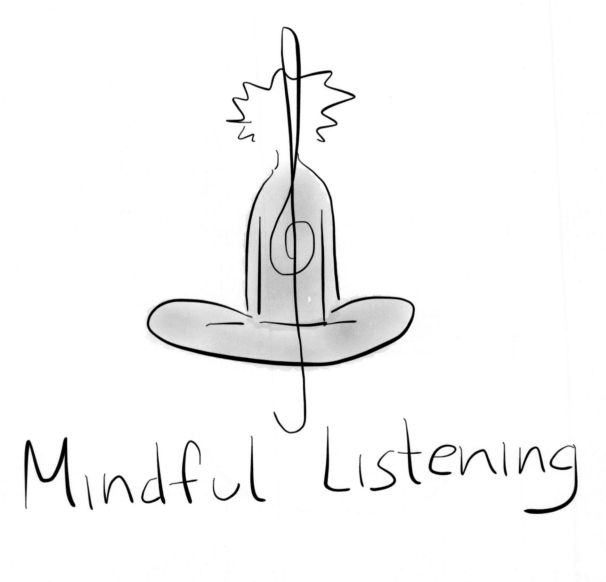

Mindful Listening

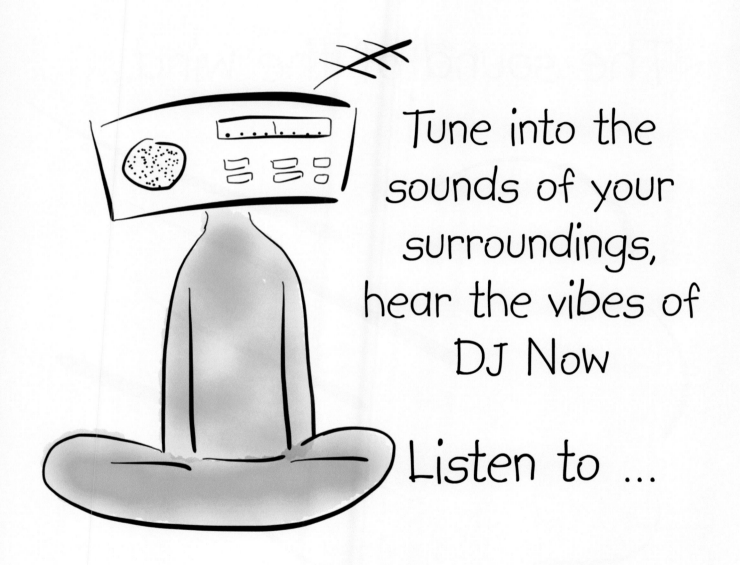

Tune into the sounds of your surroundings, hear the vibes of DJ Now

Listen to ...

The sound of the wind...

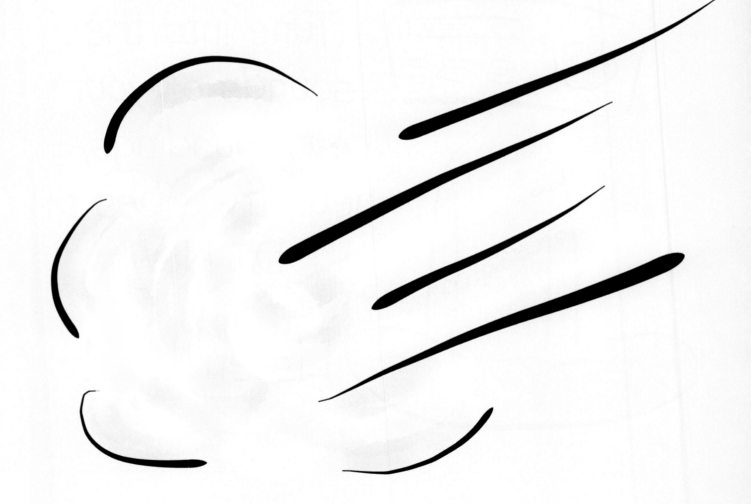

Or your own heartbeat

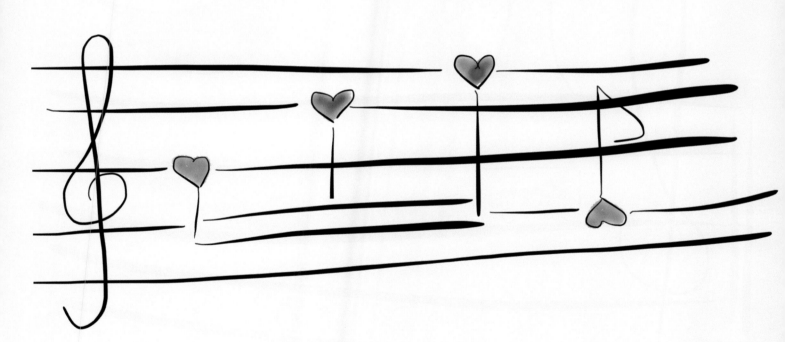

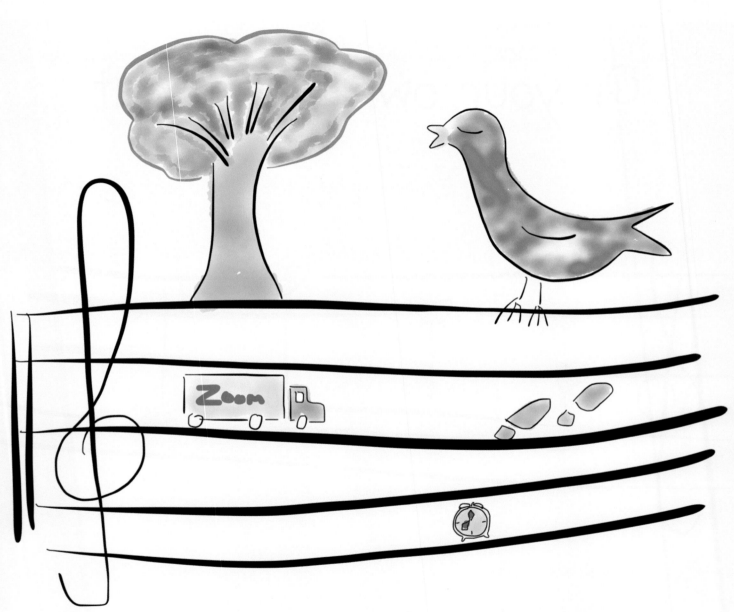

These are some sounds you may hear...

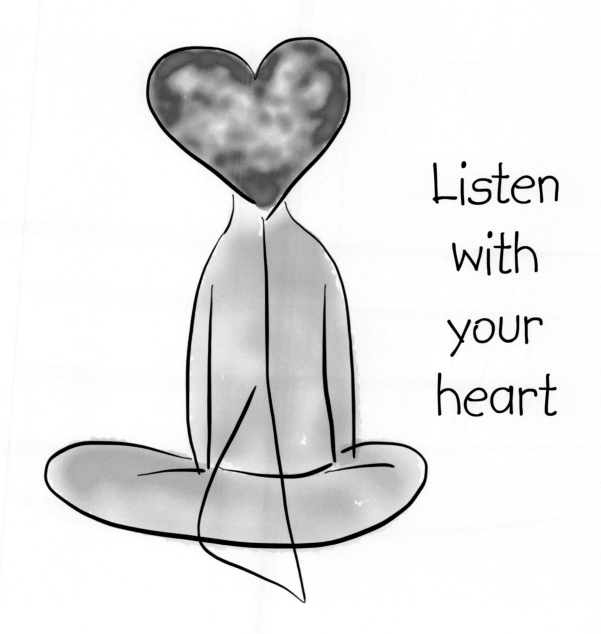

Listen with your heart

The rhythm of

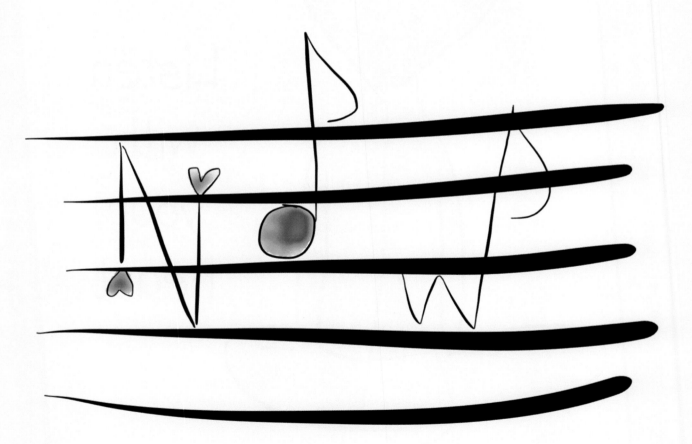

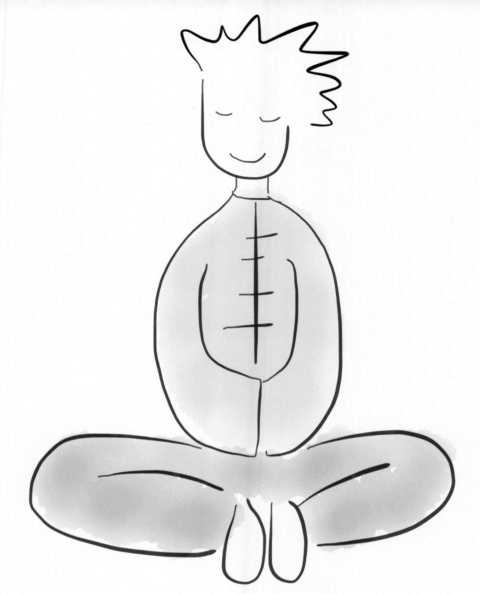

Now, let's begin: sit quietly
and observe mindfully.